How to Get Rid of Your Lower Back Pain Naturally

The 3 Biggest Mistakes People Make When Handling Back Pain

By

Kevin Kostka

Introduction

In 2012, I began experiencing back pain after working out. I tried resting it for a couple days and then resuming my daily activities but it continued to bother me and I was unable to experience any type of relief. I utilized my knowledge in physical therapy and it would get better but this was only temporary. I would get relapses. My back would, as I've heard so many others say, "my back would go out on me." This went on for over a year. I even sought out three different orthopedic spine specialists and all three had different forms or ideas of how to handle it. I then tried one of my own therapists for treatment. That's when I began to notice improvement in my back pain. The therapist's expertise and philosophy on how to treat it, led me to notice immediate relief after only a few sessions. I continued to follow this plan and was able to return back to full function and the recreational activities that I enjoyed doing previously. "My back would no longer go out of me." Because of this personal experience, and the pain that I had endured, and the relief that I received, I took a special interest in trying to help as many people as I could that were suffering from back pain similar to mine. This is why I developed this book and the emphasis of the spine in our physical therapy practice today. In this book I will talk about physical therapy specifically at Summit Physical Therapy, and what it can do for lower back and sciatica pain. We will answer certain questions you may have regarding back pain, physical therapy and treatment.

Physical Therapy

What is physical therapy?

Physical therapy is defined as the treatment of a disease, injury or disability of the muscles or joints by any type of physical or mechanical means such as exercises. Physical therapists use different means to help improve pain or other problems that their clients may be having.

Physical therapists utilize hands-on therapy where they try to move muscles and joints in the body to be able to increase or improve the range of motion. Without full range of motion the body can experience pain. The practice of physical therapy also uses exercises for flexibility, stabilization, strengthening and other special hands on techniques to improve pain, muscle activation and bony alignment. It is also common to use modalities such as electrical stimulation, ultrasound, laser, hot or cold to help improve joint mobility, facilitating healing or reducing inflammation.

What does it take to become a physical therapist?

The type of and amount of education required to become a physical therapist has changed over the years. It began as a Bachelor's degree, has progressed to a Masters and now a Doctoral degree. The training consists of Anatomy and Anatomy lab where you learn every muscle, where it originates and where it inserts on the bones of the body, what nerve controls that muscle, what the muscle does in the body and how it makes the body move and work. You learn every nerve in the nervous system and what it controls from muscles to organs. It is very extensive training and is at the level of medical doctors and their training during medical school. Physical therapists learn about pathology and all the different diseases, disease processes and what they do and how they affect the body. Biomechanics is also an important subject that is similar to physics but emphasizes physics and the body during movements. There are many other classes that a physical therapist takes during the three postgraduate years of lecture, lab and clinical rotations. All of these classes help create an expert physical therapist to treat someone who is experiencing pain. But during this schooling advanced techniques are not taught as there is only so much time during the school year to teach a student physical therapist everything they need to know to pass a state licensure exam.

What are the different types or disciplines of physical therapy?

Physical therapy is subdivided in many different disciplines. The field I am in is orthopedics. There are also pediatrics (working with kids), geriatrics (working with the elderly population) neurology (any type of spinal cord or traumatic, brain injury, or neurological disease), home health, hospital based therapy (acute care) and short and long-term care facilities.

Do physical therapists specialize? Do they have a specialty that they obtain through any kind of certification or schooling?

This is one of the biggest trends in physical therapy right now. Very similar to how medical doctors are now becoming specialized, so are physical therapists. In physical therapy, you may go see a shoulder, foot or hand specialist. You can see someone that has been trained in the spine, orthopedics, sports, geriatrics, pediatrics, or neurology. There are many kinds of specialty certifications that you can obtain in the physical therapy world. The American Physical Therapy Association (APTA) as well as other organizations continues to accredit different specialties through a very diligent and stringent process.

Should I seek a specialized physical therapist if I have a specific condition with which I need help?

You want to see someone who specializes in orthopedics if you are having back pain and in particular someone who sees a heavy case load of spine patients. They will have extensive experience in dealing with spine conditions and know the different techniques that can help the most. For example, if you took your car to a mechanic to get your brakes fixed, you would not want to take your car to somebody who just fixes your air conditioning system in your car. You would want to work with someone who is specific to your brakes. Look at it in the same way in the physical therapy world... you would want to work with somebody that specifically works with your condition, has experience in it and has taken extra education in that specific filed.

How do I decide which physical therapy practice to use? Where should I go?

As a physical therapy private practice owner, I will tell my friends and family who are out of town and do not have access to my practice to choose the company based on what their mission is and what they envision therapy to be like. You want to make sure that the visions you have regarding therapy and the mission of their organization align. You want to know if they have a purpose to help other people, and if their answer is yes, then that may be a good fit for you. I significantly value customer service and customer support. So I personally look for that service when I shop at stores. You want to know if they are able to effectively communicate with you as well. I typically look for that too. Lastly, read on their website or look in the office if they have any patient testimonials, especially ones that are relative to the condition for which you want to be treated. In that testimonial, you want to read about the results and what other people are saying about them.

For someone who has lower back pain or sciatica, what are all the options for treatment?

As you have probably heard for yourself or even seen on TV, there are a multitude of different options out there—anything from back braces, to inversion tables, creams and even commercials for over the counter medicines. Those treat symptoms and not the problem so they often fail at attempting to permanently resolving the lower back pain. Therefore, people will go to their primary care doctor for their recurring back pain. I have had the privilege of working with some very good primary care physicians that actually know some of the best options for lower back pain and sciatica. The primary care physician may have many options for you. After getting a very detailed history of your problem, they will often start with some type of imaging to help determine your diagnosis based on what you tell them. Hopefully, they are not just treating what the x-ray or MRI shows, but that they would put those two results together and come up with a plan for you based on both, as well as what symptoms you are presenting with. There is a study that shows that 8 out of 10 people that don't even have back pain with have abnormal X-rays and MRI's. Therefore, the medical doctor should combine what you are saying, the imaging results, and the physical examination. The physical exam will consist of particular movements of your spine, muscle testing, and a check of your nervous system as well as some very specific special tests. At this point, they may choose some type of medication for pain and inflammation to allow you to start a conservative approach of physical therapy. These anti-inflammatories and pain medications can somewhat help with the healing process but can also cover it up, similar to how a Band-Aid would just cover a wound. If you are taking pain medicine, it is just masking your symptoms, and you are not actually showing improvement. I believe that this is really not an effective or a long-term solution but can help short term while you are trying a conservative approach of physical therapy.

Another option is to have an injection. This too is similar to some of the medications and may have some anti-inflammatory benefits, as well as some pain-relieving benefits. This can often help decrease your pain, but again does not treat the root of the problem. I had one of these during treatment and it helped me temporarily, but then my pain came back a couple of weeks later because the problem was never truly fixed.

Finally your physician could refer you to other healthcare providers. Physical therapy is a common conservative approach along with chiropractic, acupuncture, or even massage therapy. If those treatments do not work or help, they will encourage you to see a spine specialist or a neurologist who could treat you surgically. They would send you there for a consult and depending upon your previous results with the other conservative treatments and your current limitations based on function and pain, they may decide to do a surgical procedure. Surgery, though, does not always guarantee that your symptoms will be relieved. It could even provide you with new symptoms, or you could come out of surgery having the same symptoms. Now, that is not true for all cases, but you do want to probably use surgery as a last and final resort.

Someone who is having lower back pain or sciatica might go through all of those steps and possibly even in that order which could be expensive, or often painful. So why should somebody choose physical therapy? Why should someone with back pain come see a physical therapist first?

You may not want to be on medications. Medications often have side effects that may make you drowsy or not think clearly. This could cause concerns at work or when taking care of your children. Injections again do not treat the root of the problem and often you need more injections when the pain returns. Physical therapists have an extensive educational background and training, which I mentioned earlier. Seeing a physical therapist is a conservative approach and looks to correct the root of the problem. They have a doctorate level education in the human body and the way it moves. A physical therapist has knowledge of all your muscles, your bones, your nervous system, and they are taught to understand the biomechanics behind what each joint and muscle does throughout a movement. With this level of expertise they make a logical choice for a conservative treatment option. They practice hands-on techniques, as well as specific exercises that help to stabilize your spine and return you back to normal function. A physical therapist also wants to educate you and encourage you to be proactive about your treatment. Current research suggests that physical therapy can be more effective than other options such as surgery. When compared to MRI, injections and surgery, physical therapy is the cheapest of all of the options.

Back Pain

Let's talk about our lower back pain. What is it? How can a problem in my back cause leg pain, numbness or tingling? What is a nerve?

Your whole body has nerves. Your nervous system starts at the level of the brain, it comes down through your spinal cord and then disseminates out into all the different organs, muscles and your skin. There are many different types of nerves that control different parts of your body. Some are responsible for light touch, deep touch, temperature changes and even pain. Other nerves help to make your muscles work. Different nerves throughout your body do many different things.

What is a sciatic nerve?

The sciatic nerve is one of the biggest nerves that we have in our body and consists of a group of nerves that form in the hip area after the nerves leave your spine. Once it comes out of your lower spine, it forms what we call your sciatic nerve. The sciatic nerve then runs by some of your hip muscles and in some cases, in a very small percent of people, it actually can run through one of those hip muscles. It then turns into many different nerves and runs down your leg. It is involved in the sensation in your leg and your foot, and it also helps make your hip, knees, and foot move during activities.

So how can a problem in my back cause pain in my leg, or numbness, or tingling? How are the two related?

This is a phenomenon that we call *referred pain*. It is often caused by pressure on that nerve that travels to a different part of the body. If a nerve ever gets compressed in your back, or anywhere else, then it can cause symptoms such as pain, numbness, tingling and even muscle weakness in your leg. Think of a garden hose getting a kink in it. It causes the water not to come out at the end of the hose, but then if you unkink it, the water flows again. What I mean by this is that the water hose / the sciatica nerve can be affected at one area but it causes a problem or symptoms in another area.

What is sciatica?

Sciatica is a common term, again, indicating that you are having pain, numbness, tingling or a tightness sensation down one or both of your legs. It can be associated with back pain but doesn't have to be. What is causing the sciatica is important for successful treatment.

What are some of the common causes of sciatica?

There are three common causes of sciatica, one being a herniated or a bulging disc. The second cause is stenosis or degenerative disc disease. The third cause is often overlooked, does not appear on X-Ray or MRI and is related to something called the SI joint or sacroiliac joint.

What is a herniated disc?

A herniated disc is when the gelatinous material (disc) between your spine bones or your vertebrae pushes up against the nerve or nerves that comes from your spine. The nerve then sends that pain signal down your leg, where you often feel it. It can go down the back of your leg, to your hip, your knee, down into your foot and in some scenarios it can often cause muscle weakness or bladder issues. If it does that, then you need to get into a surgeon quickly.

The herniated disk often occurs in people 45 years of age and younger. Not to say this can not happen in someone older than that but often times it is this age demographic that we see a herniated disc as being one of the problems causing sciatica.

What is stenosis?

Stenosis is related to the lack of disk height. As we age, we start to lose the water in our discs. The discs actually start to shrink in height and those discs create space between our vertebrae or backbones and begin to compress the nerve. In reference to your spine, it allows your nerves to freely exit your spine and go to your lower or upper extremities. If you have stenosis, you have that narrowing of where that nerve is supposed to come out. Then the bone will compress that nerve and send that pain down your leg creating compression on that nerve. That compression can then cause numbness, pain, and/or weakness. Remember our garden hose analogy?

People over the age of 45 will often present with stenosis or degenerative disk disease. This is part of the aging process and could be causing your complaints. As I mentioned earlier though, we do not want to just treat your X-ray or MRI. We want to listen to your history and see what happens when you move. This is key in successful treatment for stenosis.

Are there any other causes of stenosis?

Bone spurs can also cause that narrowing or compression of the nerves. Bone spurs are small little growths that develop on the bones in the spinal canal. Those spurs that touch the nerves can cause pain and symptoms down your leg. Surgery is indicated if the PT is not able to successfully decrease your pain. Surgery would be done to remove those spurs off of that nerve, relieve that compression and improve your pain level and function.

The third common cause of sciatica is SI joint problems. What is the SI joint?

SI joint is short for the sacroiliac joint, and it is at the base of your spine. It is used to help support your spine, and is made up of three different bones. The first bone is the sacrum, which is the "middle bone" that your spine sits on. It's the keystone of the SI joint. Some people may call it the tailbone. Next, the SI joint consists of two ilium or your pelvic bones. You may know these as your "sit bones" too. These are the bones that you feel when you are sitting down on a chair. The sacrum and the two ilium bones attach to one another and together are called the sacroiliac joint (SI joint). If one or more of those bones is not aligned properly, or they are not moving in the proper directions whenever you bend forward or bend backwards, then it can cause some of those sciatica symptoms by creating tension on that sciatic nerve. There are some schools of thought that the sacroiliac joint doesn't move, some believe that it only moves up until a certain age and some believe that it can be moved through certain hands on techniques. I personally believe that it does move and can be moved as this is the form of treatment that I was not taught in PT school and came across to help naturally heal my back pain once and for all.

Treating the Symptoms Properly

Now that we know what is causing our pain - how can we treat these symptoms successfully? How can physical therapy help your back?

    A physical therapist is highly educated and often skilled in the spine. They do an extensive evaluation of the spine by performing a detailed history, determining movements that make the pain reproducible and then performing special tests to determine what causes the pain. They will then perform specific hands-on treatment techniques working to reduce the pain that was reproducible with specific movements. This is where the magic happens. Not really…its science, but when we are able to change someone's pain quickly once we have all the right pieces of the puzzle our patients think it's magic. After this, they do exercises to increase the flexibility as well as the stability of the spine. They may also use something called traction, when needed, where they somewhat pull apart the joints of the spine to help make more space for those nerves and to take compression off of those nerves.

Will my treatment be similar to someone else I know? If I know a friend who has gone to physical therapy for their back, can I expect a similar treatment than they had?

All three common causes have different approaches and specific treatments. If somebody came in for a herniated disc, and we started using the treatment for stenosis, that will likely make that pain much worse. Coming in to get an evaluation of your different movement patterns and communicating with your therapist about the signs and symptoms of what makes it better and worse will put you on the right path to successful treatment.

What if I've tried physical therapy before, or tried treatment and it didn't work?

Unfortunately, that can happen. It happens in physical therapy, chiropractic care, acupuncture, massage, and any other healthcare service for that matter. Make sure you do your research. Make sure you are seeing the best healthcare professional for what you need. Find that specialist as mentioned earlier. Ensure they have expertise in the spinal area so that they can effectively treat you and be able to educate you on what successful treatment looks like. Also, a recommendation from your friend, family member or physician would even help guide you in the right direction.

Do I need to get a referral from my medical doctor?

All states are different. In some states for physical therapy, they have something called direct access which varies by state. Direct access allows physical therapists to see you without an MD referral. Now, all insurances are different so it really depends on your insurance as well. The government-funded plans such as Medicare or Medicaid require a referral from your medical doctor after your first visit or your initial evaluation. Some of the other commercial insurances, PPOs, HMOs, do not. A quick five-minute phone call to your physical therapy company or to your insurance company will help you understand the state laws and your insurance benefits.

How much will it cost?

If you do not have insurance, clinics will offer their services for cash rates that would be one price for all the services provided during your treatment. If you do have insurance, it will help pay for physical therapy. All insurance details vary. You will likely have a co-insurance, co-pay or pay an amount toward your deductible, which would require some out-of-pocket expense. Any insurance team can verify the details of your benefits ahead of time and what your particular insurance plan pays. With that being said, a physical therapy plan of care can be cheaper than MRI's, injections, surgery and even missed time from work due to back pain.

The one thing that I highly recommended is not to ignore your pain. As your injury continues to persist over time it does make it more difficult to treat and resolve. If you continue to ignore your pain it could ultimately lead to difficulty with your job, even missing work and if you start missing too much work then it could ultimately lead to your dismissal from your job.

If you are under a physical therapy plan of care and if you are hurting more than usual one day **do not** skip your therapy. That is the perfect reason to come in and see your therapist. The therapist will help to decrease those pain complaints. There are modalities and hands-on techniques that are designed to assist in pain reduction. Lesson learned is not to ignore those pain complaints and come in and see your therapist.

What should I wear to my appointments?

Whatever is comfortable for you. We want you to be able to move around. Wear something that you can exercise in and stretch in. We usually recommend a t-shirt and some kind of shorts or athletic pants as well as tennis shoes.

How much time does a physical therapy visit take?

Expect an average of about 60 minutes. On your first visit it may take you up to 90 minutes because you have paperwork and the therapist has to ask you different questions and put you through some specific movement patterns in order to get the proper diagnosis and to show you what successful treatment would be like.

What kind of paperwork would I be filling out?

The paperwork consists of a systems review, general medical history and functional outcome screening tool. The paperwork will ask you questions about your past medical history, a list of medications that you take, if any, any imaging results, any previous doctor appointments and what they have said. The insurance companies are doing surveys now called functional outcome surveys. This is data that we collect at the beginning of the treatment, halfway through the treatment, and then at the end of the treatment again. It compares how you are doing from a functional standpoint—what activities you can and cannot do and how much it does or does not bother you. It not only shows your progress throughout your treatment but also to other therapists and clinics across the county. The data that is calculated from these surveys lets us know what percent you are limited and gives us an idea of how you progress as we continue throughout the treatment.

Once I get that paperwork filled out, what will my evaluation with my therapist be like? What will we do on my first visit?

The physical therapist will review that initial paperwork. He or she will review that functional outcome survey and then may have some more questions for you about what makes your pain better and what makes it worse, and how you even injured it, being as specific as possible. The PT may want to try to reproduce your symptoms to get an accurate understanding of the mechanisms that cause the symptoms. He will do this by performing certain special tests, sometimes putting you in a position for a prolonged period of time or having you do different movements to see which movements make your pain better or worse.

Often if your symptoms are producible then they are reducible.

How exactly does a therapist come up with a diagnosis or what is causing my pain?

After performing different positioning tests, the different movement tests, and other special tests it becomes clearer as to what the treatment diagnosis is. This treatment diagnosis coincides with your medical diagnosis. Based on those two diagnoses, one of them is exactly what you have and the other one, the treatment diagnosis, is exactly how we are going to treat you. It is important to be able to explain your condition in common terms to improve the patient's understanding of their condition. Gaining a clear understanding of your condition, what causes your condition to worsen and what needs to be done to improve it will put you on the road to recovery. Knowing why you are doing what you are doing in therapy is a critical piece to compliance and thus recovery. From a philosophical standpoint, a therapist always wants their patients to be able to understand what they are doing and why they are doing it so that you can easily go home and explain to friend or family member. Someone is more likely to do it if they understand why they are doing it. A therapist wants you to be able to verbally explain it back to them and even demonstrate it back to them to show that you have a good understanding. They may even have you draw it or use different objects in the clinic to explain it to help you fully understand what is going on.

    Once that diagnosis is established, then we will develop something that is called a plan of care. That plan of care basically says what treatments we are going to be using for you—what types of exercises and what types of modalities: hot or cold, ultrasound, e-stim, or laser. Then it will also consist of the frequency and the duration—how many times a week for how many weeks. It is very, very important to be compliant with that plan of care. No, you are not going to get better in one visit. Compliance is very, very important for you to get the results that you are looking for. Lack of compliance usually leads to lack of progression of your symptoms and your treatment. It is important to follow your physical therapist's recommendations on that plan of care and be at every appointment.

Finally, your home exercise program. Your therapist is going to give you a home exercise program that is going to have some stretches or strengthening exercises included and this will help you progress until the next time you come into the clinic. Coming back in and communicating with your therapist or your therapy team on how you did with that home exercise program is very important, as well as letting them know your responses to the last treatment. This goes a long way for this next visit.

I have seen a therapist who developed a plan of care. So what can I expect? How many visits will it take until I feel better?

Going back to our extensive educational background, we use biology and the science behind the healing process in order to progress you through treatment. You have different phases of healing. In layman's terms that you can understand, the first one to six visits are going to be used to decrease any type of pain or inflammation to that area. It may take four to six visits after your initial evaluation to help to improve your motion, your flexibility, and your strength. Then two to four visits after that will work on returning you back to normal activities and function. This is obviously variable. They could take anywhere from six weeks to up to three to four months. Biology is biology, and there are a lot of things that we can do to slow it down such as diet, stress, mentality or your lifestyle. A sedentary lifestyle versus being active, sleeping patterns, compliance with your program, your overall health, diabetes, alcohol and tobacco use and your body weight can all affect the quality of your progression. There are not many things that we can do to speed up the healing process, but as mentioned here in some of these other variables, there are a lot of things that you can do to slow it down. Finally, we work on injury prevention and maintenance of strength. That is where a dedicated home exercise program will be designed specifically for you, for your particular condition and what you are looking to get back to doing. That could take one to two visits for you to be able to learn that and become independent with it.

What do my returning visits look like?

That is going to be based of the assessment of your response to the last treatment. Again, it will be some more Q and A whenever you first come back in, seeing how you tolerated your last treatment, how you did that night, and how you did the next day with your home exercise program. Then, based off of those answers, that really determines what we do next. So we use an evidence-based approach, and didactically assess your responses from the assessment and base your following treatment on those responses.

How do you know when to make progress and add more things to therapy?

That goes back to our discussion earlier about biology and the four healing phases. We are trying to initially minimize your pain and your inflammation. Once we can do that, we can start restoring your mobility, your flexibility and your strength. Then, you communicate back to us. That is very important for us to understand how you are responding to the exercises that we are giving you for your plan of care and your progressions.

I'm starting to feel better. Now what?

Definitely do not stop your therapy. That is often one big mistake that people will make. If you remember back to our four phases of healing, this is when we have eliminated your pain and your inflammation. We are getting your mobility and your flexibility back. Now it is time for that third step and that is returning you back to your normal activities. By this we mean your everyday activities such as getting out of the bed, standing up from a chair, squatting, stooping and lifting. Those particular activities require certain muscle activation patterns and certain safety precautions for patients with lower back pain. We teach you how to do those activities correctly with proper safety.

Once I can do all my normal activities and I know how to properly perform these activities, what is next?

This brings us into our last phase of the healing process, and that is our fourth step—the maintenance of the strength. This means we show you how to prevent this type of injury again in the future. The home exercise program referred to earlier will be designed specifically for you based off of what your limitations were, what you need to continue to emphasize and what you can work into your daily exercise regime. This will be tailored specifically patient by patient.

I'm finished with therapy; I've been doing great for six weeks. Will I see my physical therapist again?

Hopefully you are still doing your home exercise program. It is a good idea to re-visit your therapist for a check-up. This can be taken from the view point of the dentist and your 6 month check-up. At 6 weeks the therapist will perform a six-week check-up and make sure that you still have all your motion, strength and function. The therapist will want to make sure that you are still doing your home exercise program properly and see if you need any progressions of those exercises. Most importantly we want to make sure that your injury has completed resolved.

Now that I have done therapy, and I have come in for my six-week follow-up appointment, I am feeling great. How do I keep my lower back pain or sciatica from coming back?

Keep doing that home exercise program, moving, staying active, and continuing the progressions. Stay in communication with your physical therapist regularly. They are a great resource for you for other conditions as well. Sometimes they may give you their email or office number so that you can reach out to them or you can give the office a call anytime you have a question. Just remember you can always come back in and see them for a tune-up if needed.

Conclusion

To recap, physical therapy is a conservative option for treatment of lower back pain. Depending on which state you live in and which insurance you have will determine the cost of your treatment. Cost should be irrelevant though; as those who are suffering or have suffered from lower back pain and sciatica know that it can limit your life as well as your work. It can ultimately lead to lost income by losing your job or having to take time off. It could lead to an inability to live your normal life or participate in the things you love to do. This can have an effect on you physically, financially, socially, and psychologically.

Physical therapy is a conservative approach for treatment of lower back pain and has been shown in current literature to be one of the most effective treatments for lower back pain and sciatica. Three common causes of lower back pain and sciatica fit into a physical therapist wheelhouse and can cause long-term relief if diagnosed and treated properly. Depending upon your diagnosis, your treatments may differ from someone else's you may know or have talked to. It is important to find the right therapist to treat your lower back pain or sciatica symptoms, someone who is very familiar with the spine and understands the sacroiliac joint and how to treat it. Once you have completed your plan with your therapist, it is very important to continue with your home program and stay active to help keep your lower back stable and strong. We have had people travel from all over the United States to receive treatment for the lower back.

    Are you ready to get rid of back pain now? Call 423-777-4974 to schedule an appointment with one of our doctors of physical therapy at Summit Physical Therapy today or check out our website at http://summit-therapy.com.

www.ingramcontent.com/pod-product-compliance
Lightning Source LLC
Chambersburg PA
CBHW061231180526
45170CB00003B/1251